the Empress's Secret

the natural facelift at your fingertips

Translated and written by Robert M Klein Ph.D.

CONTENTS

INTRODUCTION

I first began integrating the practice of an ancient Chinese beauty secret, a method of applying light massage with one's fingertips to certain energetic points on the face and neck, into my acupuncture practice in the 1970s. At that time acupuncture was very new in the West, and there was a great deal of interest in what this ancient Eastern system of stimulating the body's energy grid, thereby promoting health and well-being, could do. My practice was based in Laurel Canyon, in the Hollywood Hills section of Los Angeles, and for the most part it consisted of men and women in the film business. This is an industry that places critical importance on appearance; not only is there a great deal of attention devoted to one's physical attractiveness, but to health and wellness in general—how one feels as well as how one looks.

I had been introduced to this beauty secret by my teachers in acupuncture and Taoist studies: Master Gim Shek Ju, Master Wen Shen Huang, and Master Ho'o. I learned from them that this method was used over 3,000 years ago, and that it was known to have a highly beneficial, visible influence on one's health and beauty. Traditionally this technique had been reserved for and known only by the ruling class of China. Unlike acupuncture, which relies on the insertion of very thin gold and silver needles in key points along the energy meridians of the body, this technique used a method of light fingertip massage of the acupuncture points of the face and neck, sometimes called acupressure. The resulting increase of circulation of blood and energy to the face would not only make you feel better, more relaxed, but the lines of the face would soften so that you would actually look younger and more vibrant. It was, in effect, an energetic facelift, right in your own fingertips!

The Chinese empresses employed this technique, which I call the Empress's Secret, because it was just that, a secret reserved for only a few. In ancient China, the empress was considered a living goddess. Among the many excellent qualities such a high-born woman cultivated was beauty, as there was power and position ascribed to one who possessed beauty. Of course, this is still quite true today; we all know that personal attractiveness works wonders in one's daily life, whether in love, commerce, or other situations.

In ancient China, the empress had many personal attendants who took care of all the living goddess's needs, including someone who would perform this special technique on the empress's face as a regular part of her toilette. Although in modern life we don't have the luxury of having an attendant to do our every bidding, including regular facial massage, we do have many time-saving devices that give us the luxury to be able to set aside the approximately ten to fifteen minutes a day it takes to do this practice. More to the point (pardon the pun), we have access to precisely the same beauty technique that was in use in the Chinese royal court for thousands of years, as I have translated from the original texts describing this method and developed this simple set of instructions that allows one to accomplish this method of self-care regularly.

The most frequent question I get asked about the Empress's Secret program is *Does it really work?* My response is an unqualified *yes*. All you have to do is try it for a reasonable period of time to see for yourself that it does indeed work, no matter what age you are when you introduce it into your personal-care regime. You will most definitely see significant improvements based on your age when you start the program. At first these changes will be small and incremental; within one month of starting this regime, and with daily practice, you will notice considerable improvement to the overall tone of your face and the texture and of the skin. The overall effect will be one of great rejuvenation. Over time, the improvements will continue, as this program derives its greatest benefits from its ongoing practice. That is because it is a scientific program based on Traditional Chinese Medicine that calls on the body's own natural resources for healing. Our bodies are preprogramed for natural healing and health—essentially, we are designed for self-rejuvenation; we just have to know the proper techniques to activate this very rich resource. You now hold these in your own two hands.

PART 1

How the System Works

The Empress's Secret program stimulates the flow of innate bodily energy, called chi, to the face and neck. This stimulates circulation in the cells, allowing them to create a healthy production of collagen and elastin, tightening and firming the skin, making it appear more relaxed and radiant. The seventeen massage points that are used in this program are points related to the major organs and energy systems of the body. The technique I teach here is completely safe and noninvasive, and the benefits from lightly massaging these points can positively affect blood circulation and digestion and help you to relax. You will find that by taking the time out of your day to practice the Empress's Secret, you will not only look better, you will also achieve an inner stillness that comes with calming the nerves, and you will gain proper breathing techniques that promote a more tranquil state of being all day long. So the additional benefits of this practice go beyond "skin deep."

A teacher of mine from many years ago, Gayelord Hauser, a pioneer of the natural healing movement, bestselling author, and promoter of natural nutrition through healthy eating said, "When you look better, you feel better." It's true. By performing the technique I describe here regularly, you will achieve a healthy glow to the skin by tightening and supporting the underlying energy grid of the face and relaxing the tension that contributes to lines and wrinkles. Equally important, you will also feel more centered and relaxed after doing this. What more can you ask for, short of expensive and painful surgery that may not have the inner healing benefits of the Empress's Secret? In fact, if you follow the method I outline in this book and combine this with good, healthy, natural nutrition and exercise, you may never need a surgical facelift. And if you have been contemplating "face work" I suggest you delay your decision and try this method first—you may be very pleased with the outcome.

Timing the Routine

For the first thirty days I recommend that you do this practice once a day. This will give your system a good head start. Then you can go to three times a week as a minimum maintenance program. Many of my clients enjoy the benefits of this regime so much they perform the practice every day as a kind of meditation.

I recommend setting aside some uninterrupted time, **ten to fifteen minutes,** to do the seven-breath meditation and run through all seventeen points of the program. You can do this program any time, but morning is best. If you are short on time in the morning you can do half the program—five or so minutes—at the beginning of the day and complete it later in the day or in the evening in a second session. But whether you accomplish it all in one sitting or divide it over two sessions, it's important that you don't rush and that you give yourself the loving care and attention you deserve. Making the Empress's Secret part of your morning routine is a great way to start the day. Alternately, doing it before bedtime can help you relax and sleep better. Many of my clients enjoy taking a few moments for self-care, whether working at home or at the office.

It is important that you not overdo the time you spend massaging each points or the number of times per day you practice the program. More is not necessarily better, but regular is very good. Remember, you are massaging not only the skin, but the underlying muscles and tissue as well, and too much stimulation can cause soreness. If at the location of a point suggested you encounter a blemish, sore, or abrasion, avoid that point until the condition clears up.

Locating the Points

For the first few sessions a mirror will be helpful in finding the points. After that, you will become familiar with the feel and location of the points, allowing you to do this practice anywhere, not just in front of a mirror. After you study the illustrated, point-by-point instructions that follow, you will find in the back of the book a simple, two-page summary of these points that you can copy and take with you as an easy reference. If you go to the website TheEmpresssSecret.com and click on the "Instructional Audio Download" button at the top of the menu, you will find an audio guide, set to a background of relaxing music, that will take you through the seventeen steps in the Empress's Secret program. These timed instructions start with a short relaxation session, followed by guidance through each of the seventeen points. This the perfect way to use the Empress's Secret to its fullest advantage.

It will take a few sessions to become familiar with the points. Have no worries about accuracy—you need only be in the *approximate* area of the point for the massage to be effective. Massage each point for at least thirty seconds, but not more than one minute for each point. Use just enough pressure to feel the point. Do not push too hard or cause pain or discomfort in any way. Remember, the skin is the largest organ of the body and is delicate, so be firm but gentle, which is a good metaphor for life in general. Be sure to bring the fingers to the face, not the face to the fingers, which could cause tension and pain in the neck, and we all have enough of that anyway!

Finally, I have mentioned some of the healing attributes of using the Empress's Secret as part of your regular routine; however, none of this information is intended to treat any physical ailment or medical issue. For that, consult your health-care professional.

PART 2

Preparing for the Practice

By integrating the practice of the Empress's Secret into your regular routine, you may find that this ten-to-fifteen-minute period of loving self-care will become something you look forward to each day. I suggest you establish a kind of personal ritual around the practice so that you can maximize its benefits. Therefore, I recommend that before beginning each session you consider integrating the following elements:

If you can, put on some relaxing music or allow yourself some uninterrupted quiet time. or you can also go to the free audio guide that will take you through the 17 steps in the Empress's Secret program. You can follow the timed instructions that will take you through a short relaxing program to begin with, then you are guided through all 16 points along with a background of relaxing music. This the perfect way to use the Empress's Secret to its fullest advantage.

Make yourself comfortable and keep your spine upright; you can be sitting or standing.

As you position yourself for the practice, take a couple of deep breaths and then resume your normal breathing. Throughout the practice, keep your focus on your breath as you inhale and exhale. If you momentarily lose your focus on the breath, no problem—simply resume paying attention to it. Becoming aware of your breath is an important side-benefit of this practice, one that contributes to your peace and relaxation.

Do a few slow neck rolls to the right and then to the left to loosen the neck muscles. Give a light massage to any tender areas if you like. As you roll the neck, drop your shoulders.

Okay, now that you've established the right conditions for starting the practice you are ready to begin. After the following general instructions, you will find a series of seventeen numbered illustrations that show you exactly where each of the points of the massage are located, along with a description of the point. Note that most of the points are bilateral, that is, located on both the right and left sides of the face. Unless otherwise indicated, you will be massaging both points, either simultaneously or successively.

In the beginning, as you go through each point, observe the corresponding illustration for a moment; take a nice, deep breath, and then locate the points shown in the illustration on your own face with your fingertips. You can then begin a light circular massage. I emphasize *light,* a light touch, because you want the stimulation to be gentle. If you press too hard you will break down the delicate structure of the skin, so easy does it!

Your tools for this massage are your fingertips. If you have very long fingernails or have injured your fingers in any way, you can use the tip of the second joint down from the fingertip of your index finger while it is bent toward the palm.

As you begin, imagine there is a golden light emanating from your fingertips as you move from point to point. Visualize that you are extending this light into the points on the face, all the while knowing that by doing so you are bringing light and health to your skin and to your entire body.

A WORD ABOUT ACCURACY

As you follow each of the drawings showing the points, know that you don't have to be pinpoint specific. Being in the approximate area will suffice. Use your sense of touch and your natural intuition as you proceed, allowing your fingers to search for very subtle cuplike depressions in the areas indicated. Your chi and your circulation will be stimulated by being in the general area of the points shown in the drawings, so don't become obsessed about finding the one right spot. Anyway, with regular practice, your fingers will become much more sensitive, and you will easily find that precise spot.

Okay, let's begin.

PART 3

The Practice

If you go to the website TheEmpresssSecret.com and click on the "Instructional Audio Download" button at the top of the menu, you will find an audio guide, set to a background of relaxing music, which corresponds to each of the illustrated points that follow in this book or in the chart at the back of this book. These audio instructions start with a short relaxation session, such as what I've described in the Seven Breath Meditation that follows.

SEVEN BREATHS

This is a great way to start this program, and it doesn't require any special techniques. It will help you focus on the points and the process. It's also a great relaxation technique, and you can even make it a short meditation practice. *A whole meditation in just seven breaths?* you may ask. Yes. It is amazing how just a few moments of mindfulness practice can transform us, both mentally and energetically.

Read through the following steps. Afterward, begin. You will be doing this seven-breath meditation with your eyes closed.

Sit or stand in a comfortable position with your back straight.

Relax your arms and chest and drop your shoulders.

You will take exactly seven deep, relaxing breaths, breathing in through the nose and out through the mouth.

Throughout the seven breaths, keep your attention on your breath completely.

On each inhale: be aware of how the breath feels as it enters your nostrils and fills your lungs. Is it warm or cool, thick or thin? Can you draw it deeper and deeper into your lungs with each breath?

On each exhale: feel your whole body relax with the release of your breath and notice the wavelike action of each inhalation and release.

There, you have it. By taking seven-breaths' worth of mindfulness, you have augmented your self-help practice with something very valuable: a chance to take some moments out of the day to tune in and cultivate inner peace.

So now let's begin working on the points.

Point 1

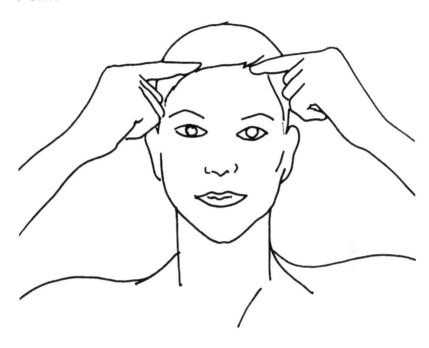

LOCATED AT THE HAIRLINE, DIRECTLY ABOVE THE CENTER OF YOUR EYES.

You are going to be continuing the circular breathing pattern you established in the seven-breath meditation, inhaling through the nostrils and exhaling through the mouth. Using steady, firm pressure (but don't press), make small inward circles. The jumping-off point of this practice opens the flow of energy down into your face, allowing you to relax the scalp and forehead. While doing this and the following points, breathe slowly and evenly and try to maintain this constancy in your breathing for the duration of the program.

This point, known in classical Chinese texts as *Mei Jung*, sits astride a meridian related to the gallbladder and liver. Massaging it may cause you to feel some pleasant feelings in your abdomen. The point is one traditionally used to treat simple headaches.

Point 2

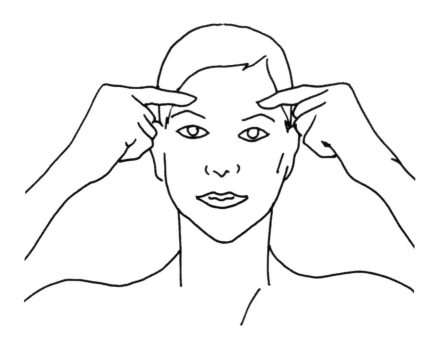

LOCATED JUST BELOW THE PREVIOUS POINT, DIRECTLY ABOVE THE CENTER OF YOUR EYES AND MIDWAY BE-TWEEN THE HAIRLINE AND THE TOP OF THE EYEBROWS.

Use small inward (toward your nose) circles. Massaging this point brings relaxation and ease to the forehead and soothing warmth to the whole face and the back of the neck.

The point is called *Yang Bai*. It is classically used for treating migraine headaches and insomnia.

Point 3

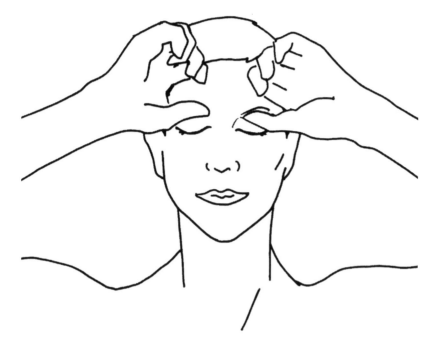

LOCATED ON THE INSIDE OF YOUR EYE SOCKETS NEXT
TO YOUR NOSE.

On this point use your thumbs. Lodge them against each side of the
bridge of the nose, then rotate them upward, so that you press up and
onto the bone and are right under the eyebrows. Use small inward circles
while being careful to put no pressure on the eye itself.

The point is called *Zan Shu*. Massaging it stimulates the flow of energy down around the eyes, nose, and into the center of your face. It is
traditionally associated with relieving headache and eyestrain, and helps
clear the sinuses.

Point 4

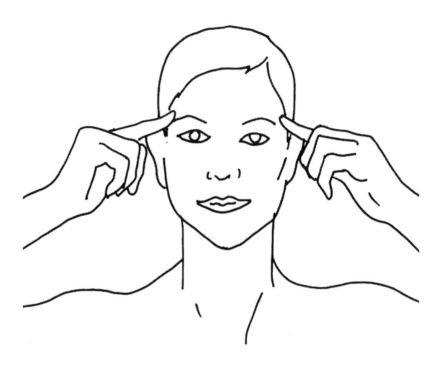

LOCATED AT THE FAR ENDS OF YOUR EYEBROWS.

This time make small *outward* circles with your forefingers. Keep your breathing rhythmic, and if you become aware of any tension in your shoulders let them drop and relax. You may want to close your eyes as you massage this point, which is beneficial for crow's feet, as it helps to fill out the tissue under which creases develop.

This point is called *Sizhu Kong;* it is used in the treatment of headaches.

Point 5

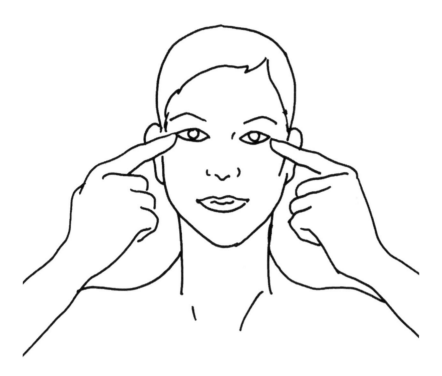

LOCATED AT THE OUTSIDE CORNER OF YOUR EYES.

Use small outward circles; refrain from pushing against the eyes. I call this point "crow's feet defense" because it is the area where crow's feet first begin to emerge. Here again you may want to close your eyes. Massaging this point enhances circulation and energy to the eyes.

The point is called *Wai Ming*, and it is helpful in treating irritated eyes.

Point 6

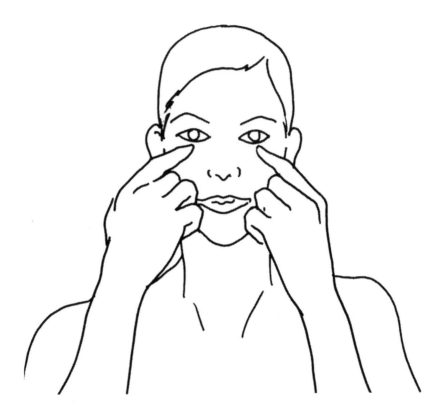

LOCATED ON THE LOWER RIDGE OF THE EYE SOCKETS, JUST BELOW THE PUPILS OF THE EYES.

Feel for that very slight depression on the top of the ridge of the cheekbones—right where under-eye bags develop. Use small, gentle outward circles, being careful not to press on the eyes. Massaging this point tones local muscle tissue and over time improves the condition and appearance of the skin below the eyes.

The point is called *Cheng Qi,* and it is known to have a beneficial effect on eyestrain and tension around the eyes.

Point 7

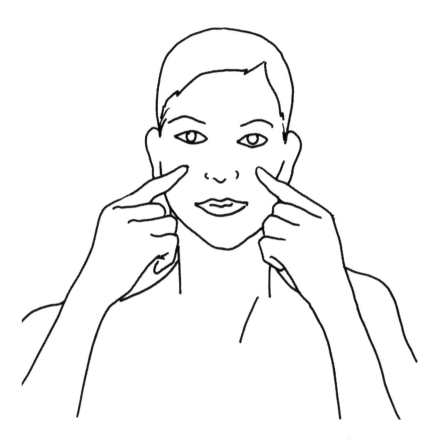

MOVING STRAIGHT DOWN FROM THE PUPIL AGAIN, THE POINT IS LOCATED IN LINE WITH THE FLARE OF THE NOSE.

You may find slight depressions at these points. Make small outward circles. Massaging these points works on the large muscles in the cheeks, helping to fill out sunken tissue and restore the natural angles of the face. Circulation is also enhanced—the rosy cheeks we all admire.

This point is called *Sibai,* and it has a beneficial effect on the sinuses.

Point 8

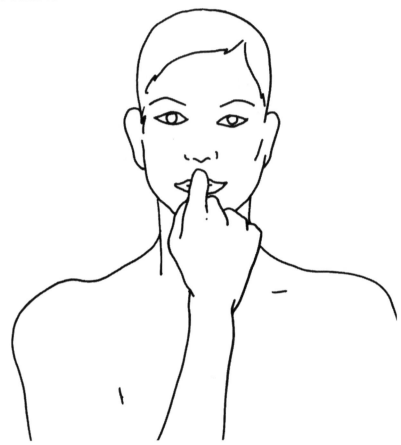

LOCATED IN THE NASO-LABIAL CLEFT, MIDWAY BETWEEN THE BOTTOM OF THE NOSE AND THE TOP OF THE UPPER LIP.

With your forefinger use small clockwise circles. Stimulating this point helps minimize the vertical lines that appear below the nose and above the upper lip.

The point is called *Ren Zhong;* it is well known in acupuncture as a release point for fainting, dizziness, and nausea.

Point 9

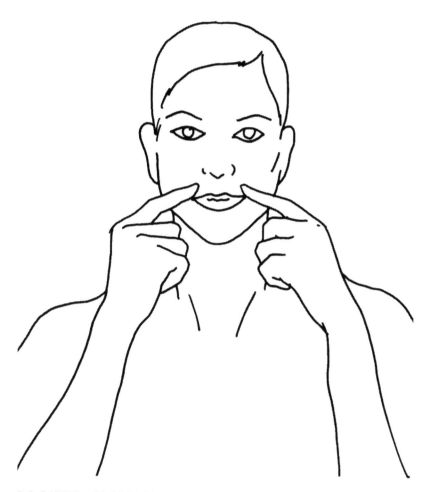

LOCATED ABOVE THE UPPER LIP, ABOUT A HALF-INCH FROM THE OUTSIDE CORNERS OF THE MOUTH.

Use small outward circles. Massaging this point has a positive effect on the small wrinkles that develop around the corners of the mouth.

The point is called *Dicang,* and in Chinese medicine it is a supporting point, used in combination with other points to achieve a desired effect.

Point 10

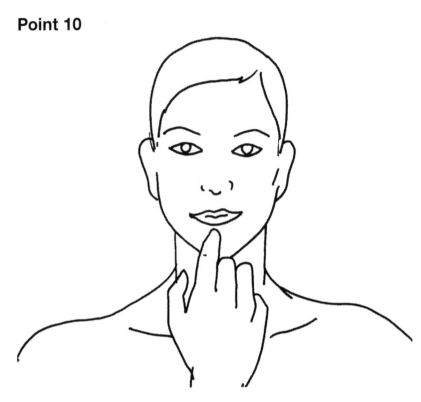

LOCATED MIDWAY BETWEEN THE LOWER LIP AND THE CHIN.

Use small, outward circles. This point is a gateway that channels circulation and energy up to the mouth and the face. This action reduces the little wrinkles on the chin.

Called *Cheng Jiang*, massage here has a relaxing effect on tension in the lower jaw.

You are now about halfway through the practice. After massaging this point, notice if you've built up any tension in your shoulders. You might want to momentarily pause, take a deep breath, let the shoulders drop, and give your hands a shake-out before resuming the practice. If you are dividing the practice between one morning session and one evening session, this is a good place to stop.

Point 11

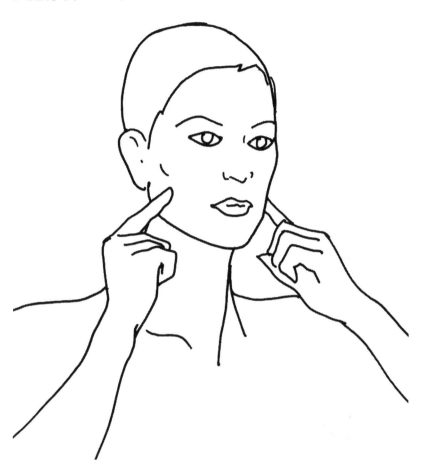

LOCATED ON THE BIG MUSCLE AT THE HINGE OF THE JAW.

Let your mouth fall slightly open while relaxing the jaw. You will find a slight depression in the center of the muscle. Use small forward circles. This point holds a lot of facial tension for many people and is an excellent point to massage to release the jaws and enhance the flow of energy into the face.

The point is called *Chia Che* and is another supporting point, used in conjunction with other points to achieve a desired outcome.

Point 12

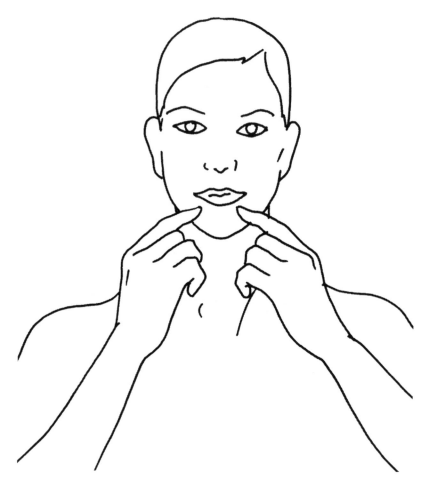

LOCATED MIDWAY BETWEEN YOUR CHIN AND LOWER LIP, APPROXIMATELY HALF AN INCH FROM THE CORNERS OF YOUR MOUTH, ON BOTH SIDES OF THE MOUTH.

Make small outward circles. This point, which does not have a name in classical acupuncture texts, is helpful for those lines around the corners of the mouth and for toning the muscles of the chin.

Point 13

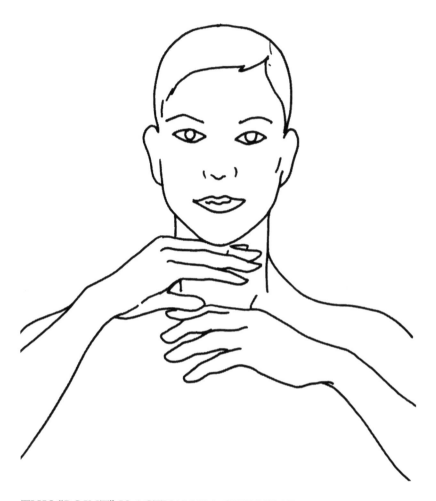

THIS "POINT" IS ACTUALLY A CHIN SLAP.

Jut your chin out. Using the backs of the fingers on both hands do some quick, light, rhythmic patting of the tissue below your chin. Pat lightly for about thirty seconds. No need to slap hard, just firmly enough to feel the circulation being stimulated. This helps firm up sagging muscle tissue.

Point 14

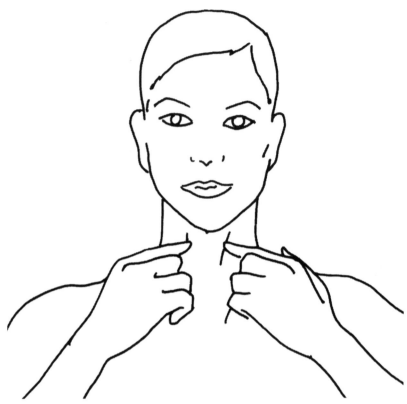

BRING YOUR TWO INDEX FINGERS TO YOUR THROAT MID-
WAY ON THE NECK, AT BOTH SIDES OF THE WINDPIPE.

Lean your head back just a few degrees to make these points more accessible. This point uses a vibrating motion—move your fingers rapidly
up and down while your fingers remain on the point. Use firm pressure
but do not push hard enough to restrict the flow of your breathing. This
point stimulates the area of the thyroid gland and tends to generate energy throughout the body; it also tones the flabby tissue found on the
mid-neck and throat region.

The point is called *Ren Ying* and is used in combination with other
points to achieve a desired effect.

Point 15

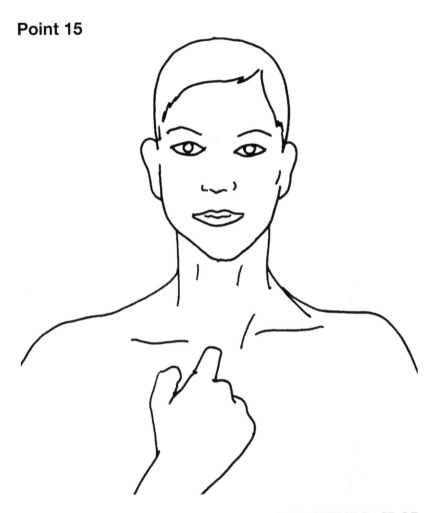

LOCATED IN THE NOTCH OF THE BONE AT THE BASE OF YOUR THROAT.

Stay on the top of the bone and with one index finger make small clockwise circles. Be careful not to put any pressure on the windpipe. This point opens up important pathways of energy into the neck and head from the body.

It is called *Tian Tu*, and in Chinese medicine it is used in treating coughs and hoarseness.

Point 16

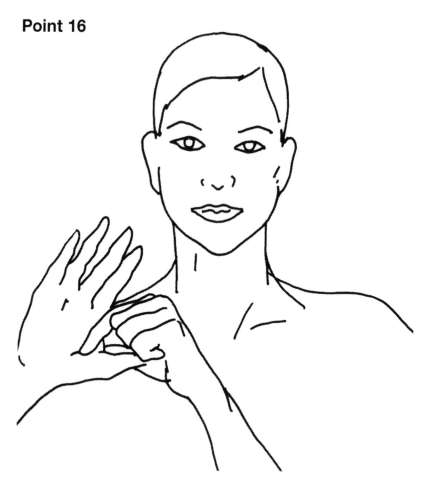

POINT 16 AND THE POINT THAT FOLLOWS ARE NOT LO-
CATED ON THE FACE OR NECK BUT THEY ARE VERY IM-
PORTANT IN THIS PRACTICE. THEY OPEN THE FLOW OF
ENERGY, OR CHI, TO THE HEAD, FACE, AND NECK, SO BE
SURE TO INCLUDE THEM IN YOUR PRACTICE.

This point is located on each hand in the soft webbed tissue between
the thumb and forefinger, on both the top and underside of this web. Using the tip of your thumb and forefinger of your left hand, find the point
on your right hand; you are essentially lightly pinching the point, with

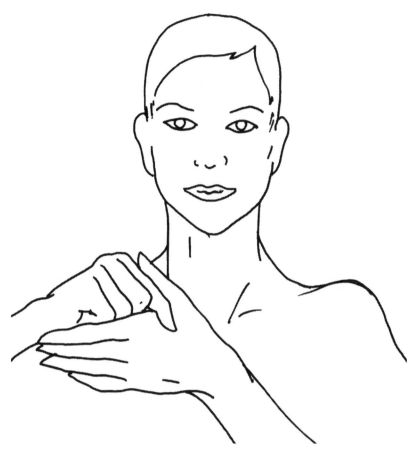

your thumb and forefinger serving as pincers. You will feel some dense tissue here and a slight depression on this point, and it may even feel slightly tender. This indicates you are right on the point. With this slight pinching action, massage deep into this space with a circular motion. Fifteen to twenty seconds on each hand is enough to release the flow of energy.

The point is called *Ho Ku,* and it is one of the master points in the body for stimulating the flow of energy to the entire head and neck. The point is considered a universal pain point and is classically used for treating headache and tooth pain, and has a beneficial effect on the digestion as well.

Point 17

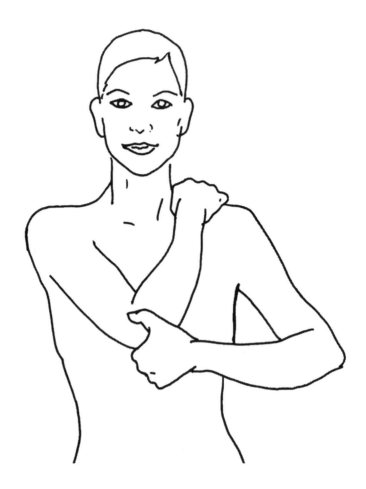

LOCATED ON THE ARM AT THE BASE OF THE CREASE OF
THE ELBOW.

To find the point accurately, put your right hand on your left shoulder. Look down and follow the crease that is formed on the inside of the elbow. At the lower end of the crease you will feel a little notch just above

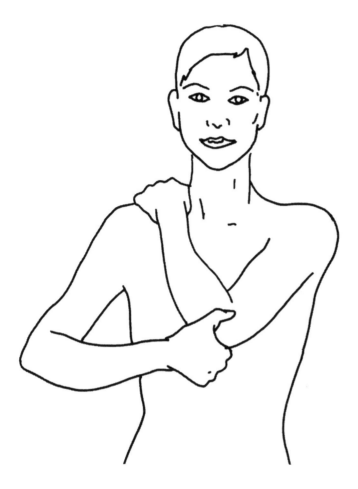

and against the bone. This is the point location. Push in with your left thumb and massage deeply into this point, using a circular motion, for about thirty seconds.

Repeat this on the other arm.

This point is called *Chu Chih,* and is used in Chinese medicine for the treatment of the skin in general.

You have now completed all seventeen points of the practice of the Empress's Secret.

PART 4

Questions & Answers

Whenever I am speaking about or demonstrating the Empress's Secret program, I am asked a variety of pertinent questions. What follows are some of the most frequently asked questions about the program.

I realize that the results you get depend on your age as you begin the program (I am in my mid-fifties), but are the results in any way comparable to a surgical facelift? And if not exactly, then how would you characterize the results in comparison with surgical facelifts?
From what I have seen in my research, comparing those who have had "face work" done to those who have taken this natural, noninvasive approach, the latter group—those doing the Empress's Secret program—look healthier and much more natural. With surgery you might stretch the skin tight enough to eliminate some lines, but the look will be unnatural.

Does the program have permanent benefits?
Yes, the benefits are permanent as long as you maintain the massage on a regular basis. After the first thirty days of daily practice, the natural energy system you are calling on will improve the tone of the skin and the very small muscles of the face to the point that you can maintain the improvement by performing the practice for a minimum of three days a

week. If you elect to continue to do the program daily, you will see even more improvement because in essence this is an exercise program for the face, and these muscles will respond just like the muscles and energy system in the rest of the body. Just as you cannot expect the muscle tone of your body to respond after doing an exercise for just a few times and then dropping it, so it is true of this beauty regime.

Can I get the maximum results in thirty days?
We are all different and respond in different ways to healing and exercise. So it is with this program. In general, the activation of the rebuilding process will be achieved in thirty days—for some people less, for some more. It really depends on your state of health at the time you begin the program. Some people may have had illnesses or conditions that would slow the process and it might take a week or so more to notice. Age can also be a factor. You be the judge: when you have achieved the results you want, then that is the time to go to the maintenance schedule of two to three times a week. You might want to do this program daily for well beyond the initial thirty-day period before going down to three days a week; it all depends on what you want to achieve. I have many clients who do it daily because of the additional benefits of relaxation and a sense of well-being—it's a meditation as well as a self-improvement program.

If I stop doing the program, will my face return to how it was when I started?
If you stop completely the answer is yes, but after the initial thirty-day period if you do the practice a few days a week you can keep the cosmetic look you want and maintain a glow of health. If for some reason you have to stop once you have begun, you can pick up where you left off and not lose the benefits. Just try not to take too much time off.

Is it necessary to do the points in the order in which they are described?
This is a very good question. Initially it is important to follow the program in the correct order. It is designed to work with the natural flow of energy on the meridian energy channels of the face. If you massage the points out of order, especially if this only occurs occasionally, it won't

hurt anything; but my research has shown that doing it in the correct order is most effective to the entire energy grid of the face.

What if I have achieved the look I want in most of my face but still have some problem areas like around the mouth or around the eyes?
I recommend that if after the initial period you find you want a boost in some areas on your face, spend another thirty seconds in those areas.

Will the exercises eliminate "Guipetto lines," those lines that go down from the corners of the mouth, as well as sagging jowls?
It will not eliminate those lines completely, but they will begin to fill out and take on a healthier, more natural look. Sagging jowls often have to do with excess weight and lack of muscle tone. By doing this program regularly you can begin to tone these muscles and in essence "pull up" the extra tissue.

Would it be more effective if you did the points on an inversion table?
No, it is better to do in a normal sitting or standing position. Remember, you are bringing tone to the skin and the underlying muscles in the position you are in for the better part of your day (unless you work as a trapeze artist in the circus). Keep it simple.

Will the program help remove age spots or sunspots?
No it won't. But it can make them less evident as the circulation and tone of the skin improves.

Can the program help an older person, say, sixty or seventy-year or even older facial skin that may be heavily wrinkled?
The good news is yes, it will make improvements to the face and skin no matter how old—or young—you are. It may take a little more time to work if you are older, but it can make a big difference and help you to return to a natural, healthy-looking skin.

I am in my twenties and want to maintain good, healthy-looking skin on my face. Can the program be preventative?

Big yes! For younger people who want to maintain good-looking facial skin and a toned face, the program will work brilliantly in keeping the tone and texture of the face at its best. You can stay with the Empress's Secret for life.

Can the program eliminate acne scars?

No, sorry to say. But by doing the program regularly, the increase in collagen and elastin will help to fill out the facial skin in the scarred areas and will bring a very beneficial look to the skin.

Are the points hard to find?

No not hard at all. In the beginning you may move around a bit to find the points as illustrated in this book, and then as you get used to the touch and feel you will naturally go directly to the point with ease and comfort. As I mentioned before, we are not looking for pinpoint accuracy; if you are in the general area you will have wonderful benefits.

Can you do the Seven Breaths at the beginning as a pranayama practice, incorporating nostril breathing?

Yes. It is a good way to begin any practice, such as yoga or tai chi, that you are already familiar with. It can be a good grounding and centering mini-meditation. Basically, it's a tool that I use in a lot of areas of my practice, which you can use whenever you feel stressed or just want to let go and relax. It is especially good to do at bedtime to help you get a sound sleep.

Will it work for men?

Absolutely. Skin does not know gender. In my practice I have worked with many men for whom looks are important. One very high-powered executive told me that after he was into the program for about forty-five days some people started a rumor that he had had a facelift. This gave us a good laugh.

Can I watch TV, talk on the phone, or drive a car while doing the program?

Well, we can do just about anything while watching TV, driving, and talking on the phone, right? But we're not giving our full attention to what we're doing in the present moment if we try to do two or more things at the same time. And if you're driving a car and doing something else that requires concentration, you're endangering yourself and others. The side benefits of the Empress's Secret program are that we learn to cultivate inner harmony and equilibrium that supports us all day long. So I recommend that you set aside some uninterrupted time to practice this self-care regime, so that you can reap the full benefits of the program.

If I have an injury to my face or sunburn should I do the program anyway?

No. If you have a sunburn allow it to heal before you begin or resume the practice. Your skin will be in much too delicate a condition to work on it in this way. If you have an injury, inflammation, or pimple on your face stay away from that particular spot until it is healed.

If I have had some cosmetic work done on my face will this still work?

Yes. It may take a bit longer to see the improvements, as surgery interrupts the meridians in the face. But by doing the program you can restore the natural energy flow system and achieve stellar results.

Should I do the program in front of a mirror?

In the beginning, as you get used to the location of the points, use a mirror to help you find the points on your own face. After a while you will no longer need the mirror; the chart in the back of this book will be helpful to remind you which points come in which order.

What causes bags under the eyes, and does this program work to eliminate them?

What happens is that the muscles below the eyes often weaken and break down, permitting fat particles to herniate through them and push outward. You see this as "bags" or pouches commonly associated with aging.

As you massage these places, the muscles around the eyes regain tone and firmness and become more effective in holding back the fat. Many women with a particularly serious condition have reported significant improvement. We cannot talk about a complete "cure," but this practice will stop the process and improve appearances.

I have a really hard time finding the time to do this practice, even though I know it would be good for me. Do you have any suggestions that would help me establish this as a daily routine for the next thirty days?

For three days keep a time sheet of what you do when and for how long. You will be surprised how much of your time is spent with busywork, work that only appears to be productive but actually only keeps one occupied. By eliminating just a small portion of this busywork in your day you will find that the fifteen minutes you need to do this regime are easily accessible. After you begin and stay with it for a few days it will become as easy as remembering to brush your teeth.

If the points correspond to certain organs and energy centers in the body as you explain in the book, will the program benefit those specific areas of the body and therefore have a beneficial effect on one's overall health?

The points that are used in the book, when stimulated on a regular basis, can have a positive effect on your general well-being, no doubt about it. When asked if there are side effects from doing the Empress's Secret, my answer yes, there is a major side effect: it is a sense of well-being.

With all due respect, you mean to say that in ancient China the men of the emperor's court did not also practice these kinds of rites?

I have not found it mentioned in the ancient texts, but my guess is that wanting to look and feel good, then as now, is not gender specific.

Free audio guide download

THIS AUDIO GUIDE WILL TAKE YOU THROUGH THE 17 STEPS IN THE EMPRESS'S SECRET PROGRAM.

You will follow the timed instructions that will take you through a short relaxing program to begin with, then you are guided through all 16 points along with a background of relaxing music.

This the perfect way to use the Empress's Secret to its fullest advantage.

Go to the website: *TheEmpresssSecret.com* and click on the "Instructional Download" button.

SUMMARY OF THE 17 POINTS

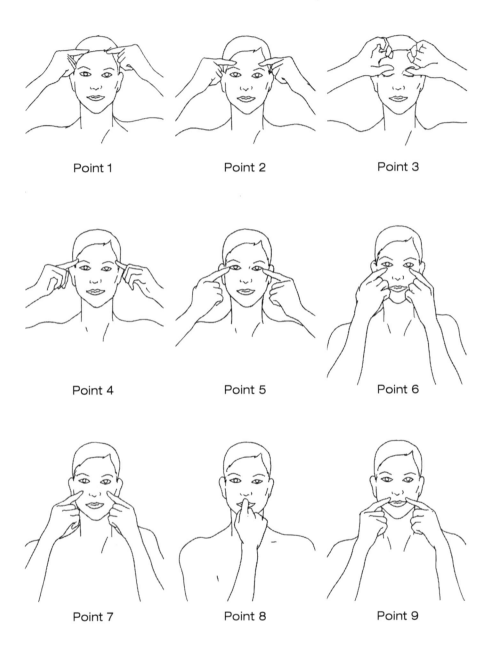

Point 1

Point 2

Point 3

Point 4

Point 5

Point 6

Point 7

Point 8

Point 9

The Empress's Secret

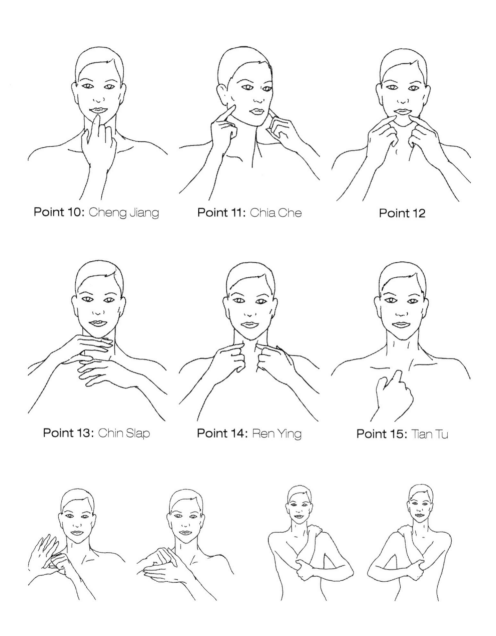

Point 10: Cheng Jiang   **Point 11:** Chia Che   **Point 12**

Point 13: Chin Slap   **Point 14:** Ren Ying   **Point 15:** Tian Tu

Point 16: Ho Ku   **Point 17:** Chu Chih

Robert M. Klein, PhD   **53**

AFTERWORD

On Maintaining Optimal Health

The points illustrated in this book are a few of what is known in Traditional Chinese Medicine (TCM) as master points. When these points are lightly massaged, they cause the energy channels in the body on which they lie, known as the meridians, to flow more freely, bringing better circulation and more chi, or energy, to the areas targeted in this program. You can think of this system of energy circulation as the body's battery pack. It is an invisible grid of channels throughout the body that allows the life force that feeds the nerves, muscles, organs, and lymphatic fluid to operate at maximum efficiency, bringing health and a feeling of well-being to the entire body.

Acupuncture and acupressure are forms of therapy that promote the natural healing of the body. The science and art of the Empress's Secret involves therapy stemming from an ancient branch of TCM, an increasingly popular form of self-care that is being used in a wide range of cultural and social backgrounds.

The massage of these points is a safe and effective natural therapy and TCM is an integrated system that has been used for over 5,000 years to treat injuries and illnesses. In the TCM system, the body is seen as a balance of two opposing and inseparable forces that we each possess: yin and yang. Yin represents the moist, cold, slow, dark feminine principle, while yang represents the hot, dry, excited, light, active male principle. TCM likens the human body to a highly complex electrical circuit. Like any electrical circuit, it must be kept in good working order if it is to function effectively; if the circuit becomes unbalanced and breaks down, the result is illness. For this reason, it is essential for chi, energy, as well as the blood to circulate in a continuous and unobstructed manner to maintain good health of the mind and body.

The points along the meridians are like small parabolic dishes; you can sometimes feel them as you brush your fingertips over the points I have illustrated in this book. These points can become blocked for a variety of reasons: stress, improper diet, or exposure to unbalancing elements in the environment. They also become less efficient as we grow older, so they benefit from some extra stimulation. That is what the Empress's Secret is all about.

TIPS FOR MAINTAINING BEAUTY, HEALTH, AND WELLNESS

ONCE YOU START INTEGRATING THE TECHNIQUE I HAVE OUTLINED HERE IN YOUR DAILY ROUTINE, YOU CAN GREATLY ENHANCE THE EFFECTS BY INCORPORATING SOME BASIC, TIME-TESTED PRINCIPLES OF GOOD, NATURAL HEALTH.

DIET: Eat a balanced diet of fruits, vegetables, and proteins. Try to balance your meals with all these elements. Eating regularly is important. Try not to skip meals or to make up for a skipped meal later in the day. Eat light, stay light. Try eating your harder-to-digest proteins at breakfast (don't skip breakfast!) and during your midday meal, then eat a light supper, and not too late. That, combined with drinking six to eight glasses of water per day—perhaps more if you live in a hot, dry climate or if you do extra physical activity—will have a positive effect on the way you feel and will make the Empress's Secret work even better.

A WORD ABOUT SMOKING: Don't smoke. It is highly toxic to the lungs, skin, heart, energy system, and the way you feel about yourself. And nothing ages the appearance like smoking.

EXERCISE: At the very least, try to walk a half hour a day, and do more vigorous exercise three times a week.

ALCOHOL: A glass or two of wine or your favorite cocktail, with meals, is not a problem. Going over these limits causes weight gain, dryness of the skin, and contributes to the little fine wrinkle lines we are trying to eliminate with this program. Also, if you do enjoy a glass or two of wine, have it with some food. Mainly, know that moderation is the key to a good diet and resulting good health.

BREATHING: Breath is pure energy: try to become more conscious of your breathing throughout the entire day. And when you do this program, be aware of the depth of your inhalation and exhalation. Breathe deeply and notice the air going in; exhale fully and feel the breath as it is being released. By training yourself to become more conscious of your breath, you will be surprised at the positive effects on your emotional, mental, and physical state.

These are some simple suggestions. There are many good books on these subjects that you can find at the library or at natural food stores. Take a look and see what appeals to you. You will thank yourself many times over.

Robert M Klein, Ph.D.

Robert Klein began his journey as an acupuncturist in the late 1960s, when he was confronted with a personal medical problem that could not be diagnosed or treated by conventional channels of Western medicine. At that time acupuncture was not sanctioned in the United States and was practiced underground, and for the most part only among the Chinese, Japanese, and Korean communities. Through a friend he was given the address of an acupuncturist in Chinatown, Los Angeles. After searching the back streets of Chinatown, he finally found the apartment of Gim Shek Ju, a Taoist master. At first Master Ju was hesitant to treat anyone who was not Asian, but after a short interview the master decided to treat him, and alleviated the problem in one fifteen-minute treatment. Thereafter Master Ju agreed to take him on as a student of acupuncture, and their one-on-one teacher-student relationship lasted for four years.

Around this same time a group of psychophysiology students from UCLA also discovered Master Ju, and along with Master Ju and Klein they established the National Acupuncture Association, opening the first acupuncture clinic at UCLA under the auspices of the UCLA Medical School in the early 1970s. Dr. Klein, who eventually went on to obtain his PhD in psychology, became one of the first recognized acupuncturists in America and was instrumental in legalizing acupuncture and establishing a system of licensing its practice in California, the first state in the United States to do so. He subsequently became a director of the National Acupuncture Association as well as vice president of both the East-West Acupuncture Society and the National Association for Veterinary Acupuncture. His work with animals was funded by a grant from the University of California at Davis, and this led Dr. Klein, along with Dr. Richard Glassberg, to develop a widely used acupuncture system for dogs, cats, and horses.

In recent years Dr. Klein has worked with a number of cutting-edge scientists to develop new models in bringing energy to the body. He holds U.S. patents that have led to the development of nano particles that acquire transient light and convert it to wavelengths that improve energy flow and circulation in the human body.

Dr. Klein currently resides in Tulum, Mexico, where he practices as a psychotherapist, acupuncturist, and energy healer, and is writing and translating books that relate to healing and Taoist thought and philosophy.

Testimonials for Dr. Robert M. Klein's
The Empress's Secret

"I have looked at the scientific basis for the Empress's Secret and am very impressed and have been further convinced by the results I have seen. This is the best way to give your face a natural lift."

Dr. Gary Richwald M.D, FACP MPH, Adjunct Professor
UCLA School of Public Health

"I would not have believed it if I had not proven it on myself, I am blown away by the positive results."

M.B., Los Angeles, CA, actress

"I have spent a fortune on creams and treatments to make my skin look better. I was skeptical and tried the Empress's Secret. All I can say is it works!"

L. Stevens, Denver, CO, homemaker and mother of three

"My acupuncturist suggested I try this. I did and my friends think I had surgery, no kidding."

J.V., Hollywood, CA, actress/model

"When Dr. Klein asked me to give a testimonial I jumped at the chance. I want to spread the word to the women of the world who want to look better naturally. This works and keeps working. I am a fan."

A. Goldstein, New York, fashion executive.

"After 30 days my skin looked amazing, and the fine bothersome little wrinkles were gone. I am an executive with a major cosmetics company and I have seen it all. This is good, really good."

Name withheld upon request

"Guys want to look good as much as women do. My girlfriend, who is a bit younger than I am, suggested I try this. At first I was reticent, but figured why not. Now I know why. I really do look younger. Thank you, Dr. Klein."

Mark S., Chicago, IL, stockbroker

"If I hadn't tried it myself I would have called bull s--- at the claims, but it really works. I use it almost every day."

Anonymous

"I am 58 years old and my face was going downhill fast. I started the program, and after 3 weeks I saw a difference. Now, after 3 months, it is an amazing difference in the way I look and feel about myself."

Name withheld upon request

"A friend gave me an early copy of the Empress's Secret. I tried it, and it wasn't my imagination, in three weeks I saw a difference. I will do this forever."

K. Alter, Los Angeles, CA, actress/dog walker/environmentalist

"I found this book delivers just what it promises, a useful method for improving circulation, health and thereby skin tone and color. Using this method provides a viable alternative to surgery. It's longer lasting, relaxing, noninvasive and cost effective. A valuable book for anyone committed to responsible self-maintenance."

Pat West, Madison, WI

"I discovered this program about five months ago and have practiced it nearly every day since. I have noticed great results! It provides a wonderful alternative to surgical facelifts—something plastic surgeons certainly wouldn't like. Still, I think all women should be able to learn about the benefits of facial massaging and exercises and decide for themselves if this method is right for them. It IS right for me."

Patricia Nolan Stein, Burbank, California

"The technique works. Not only do you look younger (after repeated use), but your face feels rejuvenated. It does work."

G. Niederkorn, Boulder, CO, florist

"In this well-written and illustrated book, Robert Klein presents a 20-minute acupressure program that will make a positive difference in facial looks and health too, as acupressure points usually have more than one beneficial effect when stimulated. It's easy to do and takes no more energy than sitting upright and stimulating various facial and upper body rejuvenated acupressure points with your fingertips for one minute each! I can testify that the facelift works just as well for men as women; I can also say that I have gifted an actress friend with this book, and within only a couple of weeks of practice she emailed me that people around her had begun to tell her that she was looking ten years younger!"

Thomas Gabriel, Solvang, CA

Follow *The Empress's Secret*

 On Facebook: Facebook.com/TheEmpresssSecret

 On Twitter: @EmpresssSecret

 And on the website: TheEmpresssSecret.com

Made in the USA
San Bernardino, CA
07 January 2020